DITCH BOOZE TODAY

QUIT DRINKING ALCOHOL
GET SOBER
LIVE A MORE FULFILLING LIFE

Written and published by Murad Murad

INTRODCUTION

"SOBRIETY WAS THE BEST GIFT
I GAVE MYSELF."

– Rob Lowe

Prohibition was the era in America where the importation and sale of alcohol was banned. It lasted from the 17th of January 1920 all the way until the 5th of December 1933. Imagine a world today where alcohol was banned for 13 years. How do you think the citizens of your country would react on the news that alcohol was to be no more? The media will have the headlines running for weeks. Business owners would be furious with the government impeding them to sell consumables to make a profit. The pubs would close, restaurants would falter and many other businesses that rely on the sale of alcohol such as concerts, theatres, and cinemas would face very uncertain futures. Pause. Do people still go to the cinema? I mean…

Moving on, alcohol is embedded into most societies and cultures. We use it to celebrate events like birthdays, weddings and in some cases even funerals. Often, alcohol is consumed on the weekend coupled with social actives like going to dinner with family and friends or perhaps a first date.

This book is titled "Ditch Booze Today" for a reason. This is not a manifesto to encourage the governments to ban alcohol. The times have changed, and we are not in 1920. It is now nearly over a decade since the era of prohibition and since then the global population has not doubled but quadrupled. There are a lot more people with alcoholic interests now than there was back then.

So, what now? Well, the good news is, is that there are also MORE people are ditching booze today than in the era of prohibition. I am not just talking about the United States of America here. I am referring to the entire world populus. Certain cultures and religions either condemn or bar the consumption of alcohol. More importantly, a lot of individuals restrict themselves from consuming the substance completely or at the very least moderate it. Living sober is the new cool.

That is why we are here. That is why I have written this book for you to read, learn and enjoy. You, I assume are reading this alone, making you an individual. Hello! I don't want you to take on the mission to campaign and reintroducing a period of prohibition in your country. Instead, I want you to read this book, take what you can from it and apply it to your life. If you want to discover what a life lived sober is like, then I strongly suggest you read on to discover just what is waiting for you on the over side of sobriety.

WHO IS THIS BOOK AIMED AT?

"IF YOU DO WHAT YOU'VE ALWAYS DONE, YOU'LL GET WHAT YOU'VE ALWAYS GOTTEN"

– Tony Robbins

We all have different relationships with alcohol. Some of us do not drink at all. If you are one of these people, then I am not quite sure why you have bought this book, but I do thank you regardless!

This book is aimed at individuals who wants to improve their relationship with alcohol. Each person reading this book will have a different relationship with the substance.

Some of you will straight up call yourself addicts. Others reading this book maybe of the notion that your habits surrounding alcohol are taking a turn for the worse and are beginning to experience just some of the negative affects alcohol can have on your life. A few of you might just be curious if your moderate consumption of alcohol is "bad" for you and are contemplating ridding alcohol once are for all.

Whichever camp you are in, this book can help you to learn what alcohol truly is, what it does to your body, how it plays on your mind and ultimately how it affects your life in a mostly negative way. A lot of the time you may not realise just how much damage you are creating in your body, mind and life through drinking alcohol.

Firstly, I want to pick your mind for you to discover what your relationship with alcohol is like. In the next page, I will ask you six unique questions surrounding your relationship with alcohol.

I have left space below each question for you to explore your thoughts and write them down in this book. I highly suggest you do not skip over this exercise but take time to realise where you currently are with regards to your relationship with alcohol.

If you serious and committed to living a sober life, building a better relationship with alcohol and ultimately a more prosperous life for you and your loved ones, it is vitally important that you establish your current position.

Please feel free to grab a pen, write down and explore your thoughts. If you are more of a technology-orientated person then open a note tab on your phone and do the same with this exercise.

Six Questions to Ask Yourself:

1. How long have you been drinking for? (months, years, etc.)

2. How much do you drink on average per week? (include beverage and quantity)

3. How important is alcohol in your life? (1 – 10), and why?

4. How dependent are you on alcohol being in your life? (1 – 10), and why?

5. Does drinking improve your life? If so, why?

6. What do you think will happen if you stopped drinking?

My Answers to The Six Questions:

Here's how I would have answered the six questions prior to quitting alcohol and going sober myself.

1. How long have you been drinking for? (months, years, etc.)

"I have been drinking consistently now for about 3 to 4 years. I'd say my level of alcohol consumption has gradually increased year-on-year."

2. How much do you drink on average per week? (include beverage and quantity)

"On an average week, I may drink anywhere between 1 to 3 days. This would result in me drinking up to 15 Vodka Soda Limes all of which are double shot servings totalling up to 30 units of alcohol per week."

3. How important is alcohol in your life? (1 – 10), and why?

"On a scale of 1 – 10, I'd say the level of importance for alcohol in my life sits at an 8. A lot of my social events involve alcohol such as meeting with friends, going out for dates or even attending seminars or events where alcohol is part of networking."

4. How dependent are you on alcohol being in your life? (1 – 10), and why?

"On a scale of 1 – 10, I'd say the level of dependence for alcohol in my life sits at a 4" I don't feel I depend on alcohol for 'liquid courage' or to make myself feel better about myself however, I do depend on it to 'fit in' when it comes to social situations. I never drink alcohol by myself, nor do I drink at home."

5. Does drinking improve your life? If so, why?

"Yes, it makes a lot of my social situations more enjoyable and memorable."

6. What do you think will happen if you stopped drinking?

"If I were to cease drinking alcohol today, I think I will find it a lot more challenging to hang out with my friends, engage with strangers at seminars and events. I believe I would struggle to date as in my generation, it seems like the common thing to do when going out on a date is to drink and perhaps do an activity alongside it."

Looking back now, I am shocked at how pivotal of a role alcohol was playing in my life. After being sober for over a year now, I can honestly say that whilst at the time alcohol appeared important in my life, that is no longer the case.

What I feared would happen if I stopped drinking, never came to fruition. I live a happier and fulfilling life now without alcohol than I did with alcohol. I know I am completely non-dependent on alcohol whatsoever in my life. I don't feel compelled to have a drink on a date, whilst hanging out with my friends or when attending any seminar or social events.

In fact, most people I meet who find out I am sober are more impressed by my personal decision rather than querying it or pressuring me to have a drink.

Lastly, alcohol has no, none, zero importance in my life at present. I know I can go out, have a drink, come home and think nothing of it the next day. It wouldn't affect my health, my thinking or personal relationships if I was to enjoy a few alcoholic beverages on an independent evening. However, even with knowing I can do that and still be in control, the desire for doing so is not there for it at all. I feel more repulsed than compelled by the idea of having a drink.

MY PERSONAL JOURNEY

"ONE DAY YOU WILL TELL YOUR STORY OF HOW YOU OVERCAME WHAT YOU WENT THROUGH AND IT WILL BE SOMEONE ELSE'S SURVIVAL GUIDE."

- Brene Brown

Growing up, I was always the overweight kid in class. In some of my academic years, I was the only overweight kid in class. This became a pressing issue for my self-esteem and at the age of 15 I decided to get into the notion of working out and eating healthily for the sake of losing body fat, building muscle, improving my self-esteem and bettering my long-term health outlook.

By the age of 19, I had achieved those goals and had gone on to pursue a career in personal training. At the age of 21, I also graduated as a Physiotherapist from Brunel University. I was now that fitness guy. Everyone knows one of them.

Up to the age of 22, alcohol was mostly absent in my life. I hardly drank at any social settings or special occasions such as birthdays and holidays. I also never lived the standard university life of going out to clubs, getting drunk and attending the next day's lectures half asleep denying I had a hangover and dire headache.

At the age of 23, my social circles and network grew, and I started to socialise a lot more. I'd go out with new friends I made in the gym and sometimes even with my personal training clients. I had a personal rule to only drink on the weekends which was sort of like the rule of no video games until the weekend and only after homework is completed that my parents used to rightfully enforce on me.

Over an extended period, independence brewed leniency and that rule started to break. I'd say to myself "Oh go on, it's Thursday, have a drink because tomorrow is basically Friday". Slowly but surely, I started to drink on the weekdays and eventually by the time I was 26 I found myself at times drinking 2 - 3 times a week late into the night. Often, this was followed by a quick shower, 4 hours of sleep and back to the gym to train clients. Here was the peak of my alcohol consumption.

At the time of writing this book, I haven't drunk any alcohol and practised being sober for about 365 days. That's a whole year. Looking back at each of the statements to the questions in the previous section, alcohol never truly improved my life. When I quit drinking, my friends didn't question me begrudgingly or peer-pressure me into drinking.

As a matter of fact, I was encouraged to go on sober for as long as I could and chose to! Woman found it attractive that I consciously do not drink which improved my dating prospects.

Most importantly, I still have fun in life. My life is more fun, happy and fulfilling now than it was back then.

I made the decision to go sober on the night of the 21st of July 2023. It's an interesting story. Two nights prior to this, I was traveling back from Dubrovnik with my girlfriend at the time. It wasn't the best holiday, and it marked the start to the end. I got dumped at the airport prior to boarding our flight back to the UK, and you can imagine what an awkward journey that was.

Upon returning to the UK, none of my friends knew this and I was invited out to the usual Friday night of drinking. We drank, talked about the holiday and touched on the topic of the breakup. I can confirm, none of us shed a tear as we were certainly too drunk for that.

It was a great night, just what any guy needs after being broken up with to help soften the blow. I got in after 2am, took a shower and lay in my bed trying to get to sleep. I couldn't sleep. During this time, my mind was being very impulsive, and I kept having weird intrusive thoughts come in.

"Well, you are free now to do what you like"

"Single again, time to find any girl you want to take out"

"So which girls showed interest in me whilst I was with her?"

You see, at this point in my life, I was in shape. I had confidence and my self-esteem was rocketing. It was during this night of trying to get to sleep so I can rest before having to wake up for work the next morning that it suddenly dawned on me how my drinking habits affected my mood, behaviours and personality. Drinking wasn't fun. Alcohol, the substance was the fun. That is because alcohol boosted my self-esteem to levels far greater than gym workouts and healthy eating could do for me. It made me feel amazing without having to exercise or eat a bunch of nutritious foods.

I realised then and there that getting over a breakup is not easy. When it sinks in, your confidence erodes regardless of how subjectively good-looking you are, how much money you have, how many people like you, if you have a good job, nice house, nice car.

A breakup will always leave you second guessing yourself.

"Am I not good enough?"

"What could I have even done wrong?"

"Is there really someone out there she can like more than me?"

Lying in bed, my head was spinning with gin and vodka rushing through my veins and arteries. It dawned on me that I needed to make a conscious decision about my relationship. Not my relationship with my ex-girlfriend but, my relationship with alcohol. I realised that it would be easy and fun to spend the next few weeks drinking away with friends. My friends would get a drinking-partner and I would have someone I can hang out with instead of my ex.

For a bonus, I might even meet a lot of new girls on the subsequent nights out from then. On the other hand, when all the fun and games would eventually slow down and stop, the real burden and reality of the breakup would have to be dealt with. I'd need to answer the following questions:

"Am I not good enough?"

"Well buddy, apparently you aren't and that's why she's dumped you"

"What could I have even done wrong?"

"There's probably a lot of things she didn't like about you, and she just didn't tell you or you didn't realise"

"Is there really someone out there she can like more than me?"

"Yup, we can all find greener grass on the other side, and there's a lot more people than there are sides to a shape"

The idea of kicking the can down the road was not all that appealing to me. I didn't want to exchange short-term pleasure for long-term troubles in getting over my ex. I knew that drinking would help soothe my emotions, but it would not uplift my self-esteem.

I decided to try going sober for 30 days. It helped.

I also started working out every day without rest days. That helped.

30 days turned into 60 days.

60 days stretched into 90 days.

90 days turned into the New Year.

The New Year moved the goal posts to my birthday which happens to be Valentine's Day.

But Valentine's Day makes it 208 days sober and that's not very exciting.

So, I went for 365 days, and I did it.

Finally, I see myself indefinitely sober. But there's a caveat to that. In the long-term, till death do me and my self-esteem apart, I plan to never drink. Although, I do have exceptions as to when I drink. My personal journey towards sobriety has led me to re-define my personal rules when it comes to drinking:

- I do not drink for 99% of the time.

- I identify as someone who doesn't drinks.

- I will only ever drink on very special occasions.

- I will only ever drink with a very few selected people.

I understand you might be reading this and feel slightly confused as to why I don't identify as someone who drinks when I can still drink 1% of the time, on very special occasions with a very few selected people.

Trust me, there is good reason as to why I no longer call myself a drinker and how this exact strategy can help you to quit drinking for good or for maybe even 99% of the time.

In this book, I am going to share with you key insights that will help you to redefine your relationship with alcohol. There are no gimmicks in this book, there are no special supplements I will recommend you take to curb your cravings or any hypnotic techniques.

To improve your relationship with alcohol, I am firstly going to show you how to improve your relationship with yourself, get control of your thoughts, and ultimately teach you the actions required to accomplish your goals when it comes to alcohol.

Speaking of goals, I want you to think about the following questions. Once again, if you want to write down some answers, please do so as this can be helpful to you.

1. Do you want to quit drinking alcohol (yes or no)?

2. Why do you want to quit drinking alcohol?

3. How serious are you about wanting to quit drinking alcohol (1 – 10)?

4. Do you want to improve your relationship with alcohol (yes or no)?

5. Why do you want to improve your relationship with alcohol?

6. How serious are you about improving your relationship with alcohol (1 – 10)?

7. How will your life change if you accomplish this?

8. What is holding you back?

9. What is pushing you forward?

Here's an example of how I would have answered each of these questions whilst laying down on the bed on that sobering night where I took the initiative to give up alcohol for good.

1. Do you want to quit drinking alcohol (yes or no)?

"YES!"

2. Why do you want to quit drinking alcohol?

"I don't think my relationship with alcohol will turn extremely negative if I utilise it for the means of masking my pain and emotions after my breakup."

3. How serious are you about wanting to quit drinking alcohol (1 – 10)?

"On a scale of 1 – 10, I am at an 8 when it comes to how serious I am about quitting."

4. Do you want to improve your relationship with alcohol (yes or no)?

"YES!"

5. Why do you want to improve your relationship with alcohol?

"I want to improve my relationship with alcohol because I feel it has started to get out of control and reaching a tipping point where I begin to value alcohol more than my physical and mental health."

6. How serious are you about improving your relationship with alcohol (1 – 10)?

"On a scale of 1 – 10, I am at a 10 when it comes to how serious I am about improving my relationship with alcohol."

7. How will your life change if you accomplish this?

"If I stop drinking alcohol, I will improve my physical health because I am not being subjected to the negative benefits of alcohol on my health plus, I'd have more energy for the gym and potentially not skip any workouts. I'd also save a lot more money from not spending any on alcoholic drinks."

8. What is holding you back?

"The fear of missing out on social events and being seeing as 'odd', 'weird' or 'trying to be too virtuous' is what holds me back"

9. What is pushing you forward?

"I am being pushed forward for making this decision because I feel that alcohol is holding me back from personal progression and growth in life. I want to make a change in my alcohol habits to illicit a change in the other areas of my life that are important to me."

WHAT IS ALCOHOL?

"SOMETIMES WHEN YOU'RE IN A DARK PLACE YOU THINK YOU'VE BEEN BURIED, BUT ACTUALLY, YOU'VE BEEN PLANTED."

- Christine Caine

There are various types of alcohol that you come across in day-to-day life. I am not talking about whiskey, rum, vodka, gin and tequila. No. I am talking about chemistry. There are three different types of alcohol.

Primary alcohols – Methyl

Secondary alcohols – Isopropyl

Tertiary alcohols - Ethyl

Each of these types of alcohols are used in various aspects of our lives. For example, Isopropyl alcohols are frequently used in antiseptics, disinfectants and deodorant. Ethyl alcohols are used for making synthetic fibres, adhesives and even paint.

Clearly, these are not the alcohols this book has been written about. When we relate the terms drinking and alcohol together, we are referring the Ethyl alcohols better known as ethanol. This is "drinking" alcohol that is made during the fermentation of sugars in grains, fruits and vegetables thanks to the yeast that enables this.

Ethanol is highly poisonous. The consumption of 100% ethanol can lead to very serious and even life-threatening events. No one is recommended to try to drink 100% ethanol. Ethanol is the alcohol you find in your typical alcohol beverages such as beers, wines and spirits.

Undistilled alcohol is the raw product of fermentation of the sugars found in grains, fruits and vegetables. The fermentation of grains such as barely and hops gives us beer. The fermentation of grapes produces wines – red, white and rosé. Finally, the fermentation of rice produces sake.

Distilled alcohols are produced during a distillation process that concentrates the quantity of alcohol in the drink to create a stronger liquor measured by alcohol percentage contained. This produces drinks such as whiskey, vodka, rum, gin and tequila.

These drinks are often combined with a mixer (soft drink) that dilutes them down to a more palatable drink which is more flavoursome and consumable.

I want to make it clear that alcohol is a poisonous toxin irrespective of the type of alcohol you consume. Some people are under the notion that red wine is "good" for them because research has shown it to be part of a healthy diet. Whilst some research indicates and red wine can have some health benefits, it doesn't at all suggest that consistent and regular consumption will significantly reduce your risk of all-cause diseases and prolong your life. Instead, it is very easy to experience a lot of the negative benefits of alcohol even with moderate consumption. You are better off NOT drinking red wine than you are drinking the stuff.

Some people presume that since the fermentation of alcohol is a process by which fruits and vegetables are being fermented using yeast that the end product cannot be too bad for them as it is derived from nutritious fruits and vegetables. WRONG. The fermentation process is only interested in converting the sugars found in fruits and vegetables such as grapes and potatoes. This process disregards all the nutrients commonly found in these foods. You are not drinking liquid grapes and potatoes. You are drinking a poisonous toxin.

Furthermore, some people believe that distilled alcohols are much better for you to drink than undistilled alcohols because you get a purer form of alcohol in the final product. I can see the logic here, but it is still fundamentally wrong. You tend to drink more units of alcohol when consuming distilled drinks verses undistilled drinks. The only difference is however that raw, distilled alcohol without the addition of any mixer usually contains less sugar ounce for ounce than an undistilled counterpart such as beer or wine. However, sugar is a form of carbohydrate and alcohol is also broken down similarly to carbohydrates in your digestive system so at the end of the day, it's all the same. It is all bad stuff for you.

Alcohol acts like carbohydrates in your body. As a personal trainer, I'm not telling you carbohydrates are bad. There's a time, place and ideal quantity of carbohydrates to consume for everyone. With alcohol this is not the case. There is no essential daily or weekly amount of alcohol you need to consume to maintain your body's vital bodily functions.

Carbohydrates are chains of carbon and hydrogen atoms. Longer chain carbohydrates are often referred to complex carbohydrates that take a longer time for your digestive system to breakdown meanwhile smaller chain carbohydrates are referred to as simple carbohydrates which are more quickly broken down by your digestive system. Smaller chain carbohydrates are also known as sugar.

Yeast is used during the fermentation process of the sugars found in fruits and vegetables or grains. This process changes the chemistry of the sugars converting it chemically into an alcohol and creates carbon dioxide as a by-product. This is why you get the fizz in undistilled alcohols.

If I haven't made it clear by now, alcohol is a poisonous toxin. There are no daily recommended amounts of alcohol you need to eat for maintaining regular body functions and good health. Instead, there are daily and weekly recommended limits which you are advised not to exceed. In the UK, the NHS suggest that you don't drink more than 14 units of alcohol per week, and this should be spread over 3 or more days in the week.

What is a unit of alcohol?

Units of alcohol define the total alcoholic content within a drink. Labels on alcoholic drinks have the term "ABV" printed on it to define the alcohol content within that drink. ABV is an abbreviation for "Alcohol by Volume", and it is given as a percentage. To calculate the units of alcohol in a drink you need to multiply the ABV by the volume of alcohol in that drink. Here's an example below.

Drink: Beer

Volume: 568ml

ABV: 5%

Units of alcohol: 5% x 568ml / 1000 = 2.84 units.

5 beers x 2.84 units = 14.2 units

As you can see, after just 5 beers and you would be breaching the limit of 14 units of alcohol per week recommended by the NHS.

On the next page, I am attaching a table that shows all the units of alcohol per each alcoholic drink.

As you can see, the more alcohol you consume by volume of the same drink, the more units of alcohol you are ingesting.

However, what is more notable is that you can be consuming the same type of alcoholic drink such as beer shown in the table but, if the ABV % of the drink is higher, then consuming the same quantity equates to a higher consumption of units of alcohol.

Observe the difference between 3.6% and 5.2% ABV beer. Just switching to the lower ABV % saves you a unit of alcohol per serving.

Units of Alcohol per Alcohol Type and Typical Volume Consumed per Serving:

Alcohol Type	Volume	ABV (%)	Units
Single Shot Spirit	25ml	40	1
Double Shot Spirit	50ml	40	2
Small Glass Wine	125ml	12	1.5
Bottle of Beer/ Cider/ Larger	330ml	5	1.7
Pint of Beer/ Cider/ Larger	568ml	3.6	2
Medium Glass Wine	175ml	12	2.1
Can of Beer/ Cider/ Larger	440ml	5.5	2.4
Pint of Beer/ Cider/ Larger	568ml	5.2	3
Large Glass Wine	250ml	12	3

When I started drinking regularly at the age of 23, I'd probably drink anywhere between 9 to 20 units of alcohol a week. Some weeks were good weeks, and some weeks were bad weeks if we are going by the NHS recommendations.

Currently, my personal weekly limit sits at ZERO units of alcohol per day, per week, and per month.

Anytime I am to have an alcoholic drink, I'd be going above my limit. One of the biggest mistakes a lot of people make with their health is that they don't take matters into their own hands. This involves an element of personal responsibility and deciding for yourself what standard you desire to hold yourself to.

I could live by the recommendations of the NHS but after considering the harmful effects of alcohol towards my body, I've set myself higher standards to live by. You can do the same, you may also choose to be a bit laxer with yourself and instead become a lot more conscious of your consumption but chose to limit yourself where you see relevant and fit.

On your journey to sobriety, you will set your own standards to live by. It may lead you to setting a rule of only drinking on the weekends or to follow the NHS guidelines of only 14 units a week.

Perhaps you may choose to be like me and to not drink 99% of the time which for me, essentially means I just don't drink unless it is very special occasion around very special people in my life.

You can also conclude that you never want to drink again in your life. This is your journey, and the decisions you make should be personal to you. It's good to learn what alcohol does to your body and to come to your own conclusions where it fits into your life if at all.

In the next section, I will talk in greater detail about alcohol and the many ways it affects various aspects of your life. Spoiler alert: alcohol doesn't just affect your body; it also affects your mind and ability to process mental tasks. Alcohol also has an impact on your mental health, your financial well-being, decision making, social life and family life.

YOUR BODY AND MIND ON ALCOHOL

"I WOULD RATHER GO THROUGH LIFE SOBER, BELIEVING I AM AN ALCOHOLIC, THAN GO THROUGH LIFE DRUNK TRYING TO CONVINCE MYSELF I AM NOT."

– Unknown

Just before we jump into how alcohol affects your body and mind, I want to outline that there are four categories for excessive alcohol consumption.

These are.

1. Drinking too much on a single occasion
2. Binge drinking
3. Drinking problems
4. Alcoholism

Numbers 1 and 2 are usually short excessive periods of alcohol consumption.

Numbers 3 and 4 are usually more frequent and consistent periods of alcohol consumption.

However, anyone from 1 and 2 can easily transition into 3 and 4 given enough time and without consciously being aware of it.

Drinking too much on a single occasion

Drinking too much on any single occasion is not likely going to cause you prolonged and adverse health concerns. However, you will likely feel nausea and a hangover the following day. A continual pattern of this can lead you to develop binge drinking. (see below)

Binge drinking

Binge drinking is like Drinking too much on a single occasion since it is defined as "drinking too much in a short period of time". A binge drinking occasion is defined as drinking more than 8 units of alcohol for men. For women it is defined as more than 2 units of alcohol. These are very low limits which you will surpass after 3 beers for men and just 2 beers for women.

The difference between drinking too much on one occasion and binge drinking is that the former is more subjective depending on your symptoms whilst the latter is more objectively measured and can be defined, determined and outlined by the total units of alcohol that you drank on that occasion.

Drinking problems

Having a drinking problem is not the same thing as being an alcoholic. Just because you had drunk too much on one occasion and experienced a headache and/ or hangover the next day does not mean you have a problem with your drinking. The games for going out on a binge drink.

For people who rarely drink, this just might be an occasion where they are at a wedding or graduation event and having a period of celebration.

Each to their own at the end of the day.

This matter becomes a problem when it is a regular occurrence whereby more frequent the not, every time you drink you are drinking in excess, experiencing headaches, hangovers and going on defined binge drinks rather than just settling for "one or two" drinks per night.

Having a problem with drinking essentially means each time you drink, you are experiencing excessive problems from alcohol that ultimately are resulting in negative post-drinking experiences.

Alcoholism

Alcoholism is the term used to a person with a chronic disease who craves drinks that contain alcohol and is unable to control their drinking behaviours. A person with alcoholism is often referred to as an alcoholic.

An alcoholic is dependent or may even have an addiction to alcohol. They may experience withdrawal symptoms if they stop drinking and can even lead themselves to death from alcoholism. It is a very serious condition that requires professional medical help.

If you believe you fit into this category, please by all means drop this book and seek further, more professional help.

Alcohol and It's Role on Your Body

As mentioned earlier, alcohol affects both your body and your mind. The most obvious affects are felt after a heavy night out of drinking. Notably, anyone who's drank over 14 units in just one night will experience a few of the following symptoms listed below.

- Tiredness
- Weakness
- Fatigue
- Lethargy
- Headaches
- Dizziness
- Nausea
- Sweating
- Irritability
- Mood swings
- Muscle aches
- Heightened sensitivity to light and sound

These are just some of the classic symptoms of a "hangover". They can last up to 48 hours which may not sound too bad but is it worth suffering for 48 hours just so you can supposedly enjoy yourself a little more for a few hours on a night out?

Tim Ferris summarises this beautifully below:

"Drinking is borrowing time from tomorrow"

Drinking feels great because you are compacting so much enjoyment into a shorter period. The surge of dopamine you get from a night of drinking is usually higher than that of many other activities you can be doing in the same period which is why it feels so good in the moment, and you neglect the impact it will have the next day.

Rather than focusing on longer term happiness and enjoyment, drinking shortcuts this by providing it quickly and intensely making it highly enjoyable and high addictive thus you crave it.

The day after a night out deals you a sense of drinker's remorse.

Ask most people how they feel the day after night out of drinking and they'd usually sight some of the symptoms listed above.

- Tiredness
- Weakness
- Headaches
- Dizziness
- Nausea

Ask the same people how their previous night's experience was, and they'd probably tell you something along the lines of.

"Such a good night out!"

"It was so much fun! I'd do it again!"

"Best night out ever!"

Ask yourself this question; is there any activity that makes you feel good today but bad tomorrow that you enjoy doing?

Initially you may struggle to think of an answer, but a few examples would be.

- Lapsing on your diet.

- Skipping the gym.

- Staying up past your bedtime scrolling on social media.

- Gambling and losing money

Conversely, ask yourself the question, is there any activity that makes you feel bad today but tomorrow you will appreciate that you, did it?

A few answers spring straight to mind.

- Not eating that slice of cake so you avoid the guilt the following day.

- Making it to the gym which makes you feel better afterwards and the next day you will know you are one step closer to your goal.

- Going to bed on time and waking up feeling refreshed for the following day.

- Saving and investing your money so that it compounds into greater sums in the future.

Alcohol in the moment, feels great. It works as an antidepressant by numbing negative feelings which alternately leads to a heightened feeling of enjoyment.

It doesn't necessarily make you feel better by providing direct joy into your life through some sort of accomplishment or achievement.

Rather, it reduces your stress and worries which cloud your day-to-day mood. It is effectively an antidepressant.

Alcohol and It's Role on Your Mind

This is where things start to go wrong. A badly established relationship with alcohol begins to create over-reliance and excessive consumption of the substance. This is the start of a downwards spiral.

To start with, alcohol reduces your awareness of visceral life problems you may already be facing. It makes you oblivious to all the issues going on in and around your life that you are passively avoiding. Alcohol acts as a vice that distracts you from dealing with matters that are fundamentally important and impact the life you live.

Examples can include getting into shape, saving money for a house, learning a new skill to invoke a career change and dating to find a lifetime partner. A lot of people who are currently living and have lived would state regrets of not having achieved certain goals in life due to being distracted. Don't let yourself become a statistic amongst the many who have been distracted by the short-term false sense of joy alcohol has given them in life.

Stripping out alcohol from your life is as simple as choosing to no longer drink the substance. However, the difficult comes in the many hurdles that lay ahead. Notably, once you no longer have that vice to cling onto, you will be face-to-face with all the problems you have been avoiding consciously and subconsciously. To me, this is one of the biggest issues that alcohol creates in people's lives.

Firstly, you will be avoiding issues which plague your ability to progress in life. Progression in life provides happiness far greater than simply having a big bank account simply because we always move our goal posts. If the goal posts move and we don't move, we feel left behind and so will are mood and sense of wellbeing feel like it is being dragged along rather than moving along swiftly and gracefully.

Secondly, as you continue to drink, life will start moving by, problems will occur, and alcohol will always be there ready to wash them away. The longer you live, the more problems you will face. The more alcohol you use to dilute these problems in the short-term, the more of these problems you will have stacked up in the long-term. Regardless of how resilient you may think you are, everyone has a limit, a point in which things become overbearing.

When the going gets tough, and I mean real tough, you are faced with two directions to take. You can turn left and drink even more alcohol which hyper-accelerate the damage chronic alcohol consumption does to your body (I will talk about this in a bit more depth shortly). Alternatively, you can turn right and admit defeat in life. This can take the form of chronic depression, a nervous or mental breakdown. It could lead to you being discarded and losing family, friends, loved ones and sadly in some cases even yourself.

Both directions, left and right sound rather dreadful and treacherous paths to take. There is however one other direction you can take which I failed to mention. Rather than turning left or turning right, you can also spin around 180 degrees and walk the path back.

That means turning away from alcohol, facing your problems head on, developing greater resilience when it comes to withstanding difficult situations in life and ultimately progressing your life towards the direction you want the future version of you to develop into.

In my personal journey, I initially turned left and found myself constantly chasing more nights out to get away from my pressing issues. I experienced first-hand a cascade of issues gradually weighing on my conscious as well as my body physically. I had let my health go and I had lost control of my emotional regulation. Essentially, after turning left, I turned right and had my own mini breakdown in life. I felt doomed and lost. With nowhere to go, in the end, I ended up turning around 180 degrees as the last and only resort.

Turning left or right will eventually only leave you with the option to turn 180 degrees and deal with the issue head on. Having turned left and then right, I would've preferred turning around 180 degrees from the beginning and not having to suffer with my problems piling up, my health declining and losing my sense of self.

Alcohol and It's Role on Your Health

Speaking of declining health, I want to discuss how alcohol negatively impacts your health. There is conflicting information out there when it comes to alcohol and its impact on your organs. One thing we know is that there is a lot of research with strong evidence that backs up how alcohol damages your liver, increases your risk of all-cause disease and can lead to a premature death.

Another thing we know is that there are a lot of people out there who like to sugar-coat things and say, "oh one drink or bottle of wine won't hurt".

Maybe, ONE won't hurt if ONE was ONCE in a lifetime. However, as a personal trainer, I see this attitude all the time where people get given an inch and miraculously, they have taken a mile.

I personally cannot sit here and write the words

"don't worry one drink won't hurt you"

because I don't know you.

I don't know your present health situation; you might be super fit and have never drunk alcohol in your life. Or you could be sitting in a hospital bed on a drip after a bender (I seriously hope that never happens to you).

However, when it comes to alcohol consumption, the negatives categorically outweigh the positives over the long term. Therefore, it is far safer to say don't consume any than to even permit a drink.

Why?

Well, far better to be safe than sorry.

A skydiver is at equal risk every time they jump out of an aeroplane. I recently done a skydive for charity and everyone I told was nervous for me - they thought I had gone mad.

Personally, I viewed it as a once-in-a-lifetime experience and thought

"What could go wrong one just one skydive?"

Fortunately, nothing went wrong during the dive. Me and my instructor landed safely, and we both had a blast of a time doing it!

In hindsight, that was a big risk, a lot of things could have gone wrong from the plane crashing, the harness separating us apart or even the parachute not opening. Should anything had gone wrong I'm pretty sure the consequences would be life-altering.

Alcohol affects a lot of your physical body parts especially many of your vital organs. To be precise, it affects you oral cavity, heart, lungs, liver, kidney, gastrointestinal tract, pancreas as well as your bones and muscles. Let's explore each of these in detail.

Oral Cavity

Health problems can arise right from the first point of contact alcohol has with you. Mouth cancer, throat cancer, oesophageal cancer (your food pipe) and laryngeal cancer (your voice box) can all arise from excessive alcohol consumption.

Although these are more common in smokers, if you are a smoker then both alcohol and smoking will synergistically increase your probability of being struck down by one of these cancers. Alarming.

Heart/ Cardiac

Alcohol weakens your heart muscles making it more difficult to pump blood around your body. Your body compensates for this by raising your resting heart rate or blood pressure. Therefore, consumption of alcohol is commonly linked to high blood pressure which increases your risk of suffering from a heart attack or even worse, a stroke.

Binge drinking and excessive periods of heavy alcohol consumption can lead to irregular heartbeats. Sadly, this is often associated with sudden death. The effects of alcohol on the heart spillover into the lungs.

Lungs

Heavy alcohol consumption can leave you susceptible to lung infections, the most common being pneumonia which in some cases leads to death.

Vomiting after consuming alcohol is common however, if you are lacking consciousness because of alcohol on your brain, you could find yourself vomiting and the vomit gets stuck in your lungs. This can also lead to death due to the vomit blocking your airways.

This is why Emergency First Aid courses teach the recovery position which is designed to reduce this risk of this happening.

Liver

Drinking excessively for a few days can lead to Alcoholic-Related Liver Disease (ARLD) which involves 3-stages.

Stage 1 is Alcohol Fatty Liver Disease which involves a build-up of fats in the liver however, it is usually symptomless yet an early warning sign of poor drinking habits. It is usually reversible with 2 weeks of abstinence from drinking.

Stage 2 is Alcohol Hepatitis which occurs from excessive alcohol consumption over time. This can cause liver failure and even death. It is reversible by indefinite cessation of the consumption of alcohol.

Stage 3 is Cirrhosis and is the most serious stage where there is severe inflammation and scarring of the liver. Immediately stopping drinking can improve health outcomes and life expectancy. However, a person at this stage who continues to drink is at a 50% risk of death over the subsequent 5 years.

Kidneys

As mentioned earlier, alcohol leads to high blood pressure. The kidneys are responsible for filtering the blood and excessive alcohol consumption can lead to chronic kidney disease which make require treatment such as dialysis or even a kidney transplant dependent on the severity.

Gastrointestinal Tract

Alcohol is inflammatory to the body. Excessive consumption can lead to irritation and inflammation of the lining in your intestines leading to ulcers. This affects your body's ability to absorb nutrients and vitamins. In severe cases it can lead to intestinal and colon cancers.

Pancreas

Excessive drinking can also lead to the inflammation of your pancreas. You may experience fever, vomiting and unintentional weight loss. This can also lead to death.

Bones

Alcohol affects your body's ability to absorb calcium from the gastrointestinal tract as the lining is inflamed. A lack of calcium leads to weak and thin bones. This can also lead to increase susceptibility to fractures and breaking of bones. In some cases, it can lead to the development of osteoarthritis.

Fertility

Excessive and long-term alcohol consumption can lead to fertility issues in both men and women.

Drinking during pregnancy is also associated with damage to the unborn baby's development.

WHY YOU STRUGGLE TO STOP DRINKING

'FEAR HAS TWO MEANINGS; "FORGET EVERYTHING AND RUN" OR "FACE EVERYTHING AND RISE."

THE CHOICE IS YOURS.'

– Zig Ziglar

Alcohol and Drugs:

Alcohol is commonly known to be an addictive substance. I don't like using the term substance when referring to alcohol because, it's a drug which is why earlier in the book when we spoke about the era of prohibition it was banned.

Many years ago, cocaine was legally being used as an additive in a popular sugary cola drink. It was banned, and never again has the sale of cocaine in any over-the-counter format been legalised.

Cocaine has a lot of harmful effects on your body and mind. So does alcohol. Both are drugs in their own capacity. Even caffeine is a form of drug. The differentiator between why some of these are legal to consume and why others are illegal to consume is determined by the overall impact the drug has on you and to society.

Isolated drug use doesn't often lead to severe, adverse and life-threating events. Nor does going to the gym for one workout in a lifetime give you the dream body you've always wanted.

Everything has a compound affect and consistency is key when it comes to experiencing the positive benefits of working out as well as the negative impacts that drugs, including alcohol can have on your life.

To the average person who drinks both coffee and alcohol, they are more likely to drink coffee more regularly than they do caffeine. That is because the negative effects of caffeine consumption such as the post-coffee slump tend to be less intense and last shorter than the negative effects of alcohol – headache, nausea, weakness etc.

It is easier to drink coffee every day and maintain adequate functioning to be present at home with family, go to work and do a good job as well as keeping up with your hobbies. However, this is a lot more difficult if you were to drink every day.

Although, some people do drink every day and to some degree, continue to keep up with their life. These are alcoholics who have become dependent on alcohol to the point whereby withdrawal of it can lead to death as mentioned earlier.

Dopamine

One of the reasons you therefore struggle to stop drinking regardless of you are an alcoholic or not is because it is addictive. When you consume alcohol, it releases the neuromodulator called dopamine in your brain. Dopamine is brain's reward chemical. It is released to reward pleasurable behaviour. Notice I say pleasurable behaviour and not good behaviour. That's because dopamine is released whenever something makes you feel good but the act of what you are doing may not necessarily be good for you.

Examples of things that release dopamine include.

- Eating chocolate
- Eating ultra-processed foods
- Drinking coffee
- Drinking alcohol
- Watching TV
- Reading books
- Scrolling through social media
- Reading books
- Walking
- Exercise
- Sex

As you can see, some of these activities have obvious positive health benefits, some have negative health benefits, and some can have either positive or negative depending on the context.

If it is pleasurable, dopamine is being released. What is interesting is that dopamine is mainly released in the run up to activities such as waiting for your fast-food order, selecting and loading a film on Netflix, scrolling through social media to find a reel and getting ready to go out on a night of drinking.

Passive Peer Pressure

During New Year's 2024, I went out with my friends to a club, all of whom were drinking. I had a great time without drinking alcohol. The reason is that it's the event itself that releases the dopamine, not the alcohol. However, when you combine a social event with alcohol your brain is beginning to associate the release of dopamine with alcohol rather than the social aspect of meeting up with your friends.

This association between alcohol and dopamine can lead you down a bad spiral overtime whereby you seek drinking alcohol over socialising. But, to drink alcohol, you want someone to drink with therefore, you find any excuse to go out with anyone to have a drink. When you compound this over time, you create a greater pool of drinking buddies. Each one of you wants to go out but you just want to go out to drink rather than to hang out.

Here is where the peer-pressure aspect of drinking alcohol begins to develop. Now that you have more people to go out drinking with, you will be subjected to more invitations for dinking occasions. Saying no to one event this coming weekend is easy, but saying no subsequently to three, four or even five groups of friends will require a lot more restraint which makes it a lot harder to resist and then again, your brain will tell you the following.

"Oh, go on, a few drinks won't hurt".

This is how alcohol, a relatively harmless substance when consumed in isolated events can turn into a bigger problem by introducing itself as a by habit in your life. It all starts with you forming an association in your brain between the consumption of alcohol and the release of dopamine.

As time goes by, you need more alcohol to release the same amount of dopamine which can either be satisfied by consuming more in a single session (binge drinking) or by drinking more frequently (having a drinking problem).

Breaking up the neurochemical association is easier said than done however, it's not the only factor we need to focus on. We will discuss how to do this a little later in the book.

I think for most people, what makes quitting alcohol so hard is not the dependency of alcohol releasing the feel-good chemical of dopamine in the brain and giving you an immediate sense of being pleasured.

Instead, it is the social circles you form around drinking alcohol which creates a passive sense of peer-pressure to drink when you meet up with family and friends.

Think about the last five times you met up with your friends. How many of those times was alcohol involved?

I'm not saying your friends are bad people and are to blame for why you drink alcohol. They are equally as oblivious to this association as you may have been prior to reading this book.

I know I never realised that I would go out to drink alcohol and use my meeting my friends as an excuse to do so. It was only until I found myself lying in bed after being out drinking with my friends the day after my breakup that I came to realise this.

Life Problems

Lastly, a lot of people drink alcohol to soothe themselves. As already mentioned, the release of dopamine that comes from drinking alcohol makes you feel good. After a long day at work, cracking open a bottle of beer or pouring yourself a glass of wine can seem like a nice reward. It is even more pleasurable after a hard or even stressful day at work.

The more tired, anxious, or stressed you might find yourself, the greater the relief from these emotions you will get from drinking alcohol. This is because the release of dopamine offsets these feeling and emotions.

When you touch a hot stove, you don't necessarily jump and pull your hand away because it is burning. Instead, your temperature sensors in your hand detect a massive change in temperature from room temperature to that of the hot stove. The same goes for when you place your hand in a bucket of ice-cold water.

When it comes to your feelings and emotions, you don't have a gauge of 1 – 10 to rate how happy or sad you feel. Instead, a lot of the emotions you feel are changes in your level of happiness or sadness.

You can see this being played out in your life in many ways. Imagine you have a well-paying job; your mortgage is paid off and you have savings. Suddenly you drive your car over some glass and two of your tyres are punctured, how would that impact your mood? You might become 1% poorer because of scenario but I'm sure your difference in mood will be greater than 1%.

The same goes the other way round. Imagine you are going through a bad period in life – you lost your job; you are struggling to find another one and your savings are dipping. On a night out you meet who you think is the love of your life and suddenly, all your problems no longer seem to matter, and your level of happiness has dramatically improved despite still being jobless and unable to find a new job.

Alcohol has the same effect on your psychology but in an artificial way. The release of dopamine when you spend time with your newly found lover is like the release of dopamine you experience from drinking alcohol. Just how you may become less bothered with searching for a new job after spending time with your new partner, the same happens after a night out of drinking alcohol. Your motivation for progression in life diminishes.

This is the last reason you struggle to quit alcohol. The substance gives you an artificial feeling that life is good and that there is nothing to worry about. This is a great feeling; I cannot contest that. However, for this feeling to persist the cause of it must remain – the newly found partner or in this case, the alcohol. You will need more and more alcohol to get the same release of dopamine to sustain this feeling.

If you were to strip away alcohol from your life, the feeling of "Life's good!" will diminish and you will have to come face-to-face with your true emotions and any of the unsolved problems you have in your life. This is hard. In fact, it is very hard. However, anything that is hard is worth doing and just because it is hard, it doesn't make it impossible.

In the next session, I'm going to discuss how removing alcohol from your life will provide you dramatic benefits in terms of your physical health, your mind and your mental health.

THE BENEFITS OF QUITTING ALCHOL

"ALCOHOLISM IS TO GIVE UP EVERYTHING FOR ONE THING. SOBRIETY IS TO GIVE UP ONE THING FOR EVERYTHING."

– Unknown

Body Composition Health Benefits

As a personal trainer, I often get asked the following question quite regularly by clients and followers on my social media.

"What is the best alcoholic drink to consume?"

When it comes to your health and fitness especially if you are conscious about your weight, muscle mass and physical appearance, the answer is NONE whatsoever.

People will often believe the misconception that any beer you drink will automatically be stored as body fat right in your belly.

This simply is not true.

Your body cannot burn or store body fat in specific areas depending on what you consume or exercises you perform respectively. Simply put, your body can only store excess calories and the key word there is excess.

Suppose you require 2,000 calories to maintain your bodily functions. One day you decide to eat 1,740 calories before going out and having two, double vodka soda limes. Each shot of vodka has about 65 calories, a double serving is 130 calories and two of these would have 260 calories total. Well 1,740 plus 260 calories equal 2,000 calories. You will neither gain nor lose weight because of the alcohol consumed.

However, suppose you instead consumed five pints of beer each containing 208. Let's do the math.

Food calories: 1,750

Beer calories: 208 * 5 = 1040

Total calories = 2,890

You would now be over your daily maintenance calories by 890. Given each pound of body fat contains 3,500 calories, this would mean the extra beers would have caused a quarter pound of fat being stored on your body.

This is not much when you look at it separately however, if you did this once a week, every week for a year it would equate to 13 pounds of excess fat being stored, about a stone!

Here's the problem with drinking…

You get a double-whammy of negative health benefits. Firstly, if you don't realise how much you are drinking, you will be unaware of the empty calories you are consuming. There is no nutritional value derived from drinking alcohol. Excess body-fat is inflammatory to your body and increases your risk of many diseases from high blood pressure, heart attack, stroke, cancer, diabetes… the list goes on.

This is in addition to all the negative health consequences listed in the chapter 'Your Body and Mind on Alcohol'.

Put simply, if you care about your body composition and physical appearance, it is best to stay away from any alcohol consumption.

Sleep Health Benefits

Alcohol is metabolized in your liver at a rate of about 1 unit of alcohol per hour. Most people consume alcohol late in the night, close to bedtime. Drink, especially late in the night will create sleep problems the very basic being a tendency to get up in the middle of the night to urinate.

Alcohol is a sedative meaning it can help put you to sleep. During the early parts of the night when you have alcohol in your system, you are likely to experience longer periods of deep sleep. However, later into the night after your body has finished metabolizing the alcohol, you will experience lighter sleep, which is often met with frequently waking up, struggling to get back to sleep which ultimately leads to low-quality sleep and a feeling of tiredness and lethargy during the subsequent day or days.

Removing alcohol from your life will usually result in overall better sleep quality. The more you usually drink, once you stop, this benefit will become more apparent. Not only that, but you will also find yourself being more alert, functional and productive throughout the day.

A lack of sleep can also lead to increased hunger and cravings, therefore removing alcohol and improving your sleep quality can have these urges for more food subside which also helps to improve your body composition as mentioned in the point before.

Vital Organ Health Benefits

Oral Cavity

Reducing your consumption of alcohol will also reduce your risk of cancers associated with your oral cavity such as mouth, throat, oesophageal and, laryngeal.

Moreover, by not consuming alcohol you are less susceptible to vomiting which can irritate your throat lining due to the stomach acid that is brought up during a spelling of vomiting. This also reduces your risk of dying from suffocating on your own vomit after a heavy night of drinking.

Heart/ Cardiac

By reducing your consumption of alcohol, you will stop the weakening of your heart muscles which it causes. This can help to improve your resting heart rate as well as your blood pressure. You also reduce your risk of irregular heartbeats which can lead to death.

Lungs

Drinking less alcohol will also reduce your susceptibility to lung infections. As mentioned earlier, you are at reduce risk of alcohol-induced vomiting which can block your airways and lead to a sudden death.

Consuming less alcohol will also make you feel more energised which may incline you to become more physically active. This physical activity can improve your cardiovascular system by reducing resting heart rate, improving blood pressure and your lung capacity, all of which reduces your risk of cardiovascular and lung disease.

Liver

Eliminating alcohol consumption gives your liver a chance to repair itself to maintain good liver function. This will improve your body's ability to filter the blood of harmful substances and to produce bile – a fluid that helps in the digestion of fats.

Kidneys

Reducing alcohol consumption helps to improve your blood pressure which also helps to improve kidney function reducing the risk of chronic kidney disease.

Gastrointestinal Tract

Since alcohol has an inflammatory impact on your organs especially your GI tract. Reducing your consumption will lead to better absorption of nutrients and vitamins which will improve a vast array of your bodily functions as well as reducing your risk of intestinal and colon cancers.

Pancreas

Excessive drinking can also lead to the inflammation of your pancreas. However, reducing your consumption of alcohol reduces your changes of experiencing fever, vomiting and unintentional weight loss due to damaging your liver.

Bones

I mentioned before that alcohol reduces your GI tract's ability to absorb nutrients. Ceasing the consumption of alcohol will help you to absorb more calcium from the foods you consume resulting in stronger bones, less susceptibility of break or fractures and a reduced risk of osteoarthritis.

Fertility

Drinking less will improve your fertility whether you are a male or female. More significantly, pregnant women who cease drinking will reduce the risk of damage to the unborn baby's development whilst in the womb,

Benefits of Quitting Alcohol on Your Mind

After a few drinks on a night out, a lot of us have woken up the following day in dismay as we begin to replay the events that we remember from the previous night. I'm sure if you are reading this book, you may remember an instance where you may have said or done something to someone during a night out of drinking that you regretted the following day. I can put my hands up and say that I am guilty of it too.

Alcohol reduces your inhibitions meaning, it makes you less self-conscious and relaxed in your thinking. This can make alcohol useful for loosening yourself up when confronted with new and anxiety-inducing social situations and encounters. However, this benefit quickly turns into a negative once you consume too much alcohol and begin to say and do things that you regret.

As you can see, immediately upon quitting alcohol you will no longer be faced with the regret and guilt of your untamed actions during drinking events. This can save you a lot of embarrassment by not saying things you regret. It can save you money by not breaking items or losing and misplacing your possessions. A lot of cases have also been reported where punters have had their drinks spiked to wake up the next day with the phone, wallet and jewellery nowhere to be found and sadly, stollen. Lastly, it can also save lives.

Lastly, lot of deaths from road traffic accidents occur due to drink drivers. The reduction of inhibitions fuelled by alcohol lead to an unrealistic sense of self-ability which gives a lot of drinkers the false sense that they are fit to drive. They are nowhere near the legal drinking limit and pose a threat to their own life and the public's when they get behind the wheel of a vehicle. Quitting drinking may not just save your life but many others.

Mental Health Benefits of Quitting Alcohol

I have spoken extensively about the role of alcohol and how it releases vast amounts of dopamine in your brain. This release of dopamine makes you feel good, so good that you forget about your problems. However, the absence of alcohol leaves you feeling sad, upset and even depressed because when you are not drinking alcohol, you don't get the same spike in dopamine when doing day-to-day activities. This makes is harder to seek joy from the regular activities and hobbies you have in life, and it becomes increasingly more difficult to be present to the moments that truly matter in life.

Removing alcohol from your life can have tremendous benefits for your mental health. To start with, you will start to feel joy again in the activities you used to enjoy. These can be things as simple as watching TV to playing a sport or even spending time with your family, friends, spouse and children. You will start to seek more real joy from an activity rather than fake enjoyment from a substance.

In addition to this, you will no longer have alcohol clouding your self-consciousness. This will bring to the surface any problems in life that you have been putting off. This may sound scary, however, by exercising discipline to completely quit drinking alcohol you will become a more resilient version of yourself. This same resilience will help you to address the problems in your life that you have been unconsciously avoiding while you were previously being held hostage by alcohol.

As time goes by, you will deal with your problems one-by-one, seek joy in more meaningful activities and ultimately discover a new, sober and happier version of yourself.

THE METHOD FOR QUITTING ALCOHOL FOR GOOD

"YOU ARE SELFISH IN YOUR ADDICITON, SO YOU HAVE TO BE EVEN MORE SELFISH IN YOUR SOBRIETY"

– Tom Woodman

Lifestyle Change

Quitting drinking is easier said than done.

Please don't be disheartened when I say that.

It's good news.

A lot of the time people love to scapegoat progressive action by claiming it's far easier to speak about it than it is to do it. Whilst it is true that talking the talk is easier than walking the walk, you can still speak yourself into existence.

If by now this book has not left you feeling repulsed by the idea of consuming another alcoholic drink, you may just need a little more nudging or guidance to tip you over the edge into sobriety.

I want you to think about sobriety as a commitment, a way of living rather than a process to undergo. Becoming sober doesn't require you to follow daily steps each day for a prolonged period like how you would follow a workout and nutrition plan when trying to reach your fitness goals. Instead, becoming sober takes a single decision that happens within a single day.

If that sounds easier said than done, then please continue reading because I'm going to show you that it is easier done than said.

When most people state, "it's easier said than done", they're merely describing in the literal sense that it is easier to say you are going to quit than KEEP UP with quitting. Quitting is easy, keeping up with the act of quitting is hard. But before you keep up with your commitment to quit, you must first, quit.

Keeping up with your commitment to quit alcohol requires some of the following actions.

- Locking away all your alcohol
- Throwing away all your alcohol
- Saying no to many social events
- Attending alcoholics anonymous
- Not taking any money or credit cards to social events

However, the act of deciding to quit is much simpler than that. When you decide to quit, you must make one decision - the decision to just stop drinking.

I'm going to ask you a few questions shortly and all I ask of you is that you say "yes" to each of the following.

"Do you want to quit alcohol?"

"Are you ready to quit alcohol?"

"Are you going to quit alcohol today?"

If you answered yes to each of the three questions, congratulations, you've now quit alcohol! Now comes the slightly harder part, the part where you must keep up with quitting alcohol. This is the challenging part because you are in uncharted territory. Once you quit drinking, you never know how other people are going to take your decision, if you will feel tempted to drink again, what you will do when you are in a social setting and there is alcohol surrounding you etc. etc.

Here's the part where I make the transition process smoother for you. I am going to help to train you up to refrain from relapsing on your decision to quit drinking and ultimately to keep up with quitting alcohol and staying sober.

I am now going to ask you a series of eight unique questions. Each one will be regarding your alcohol habits. Now that you have committed yourself to being sober, the answers to each question should be straight forward. I have left some space below each question for you to write down your answers. Ready?

1. Do you drink after a weekday at work?

2. Do you drink on weekends?

3. How many days a week do you drink?

4. What time of day do you usually drink?

5. What do you drink?

6. How much do you drink?

7. How do you feel when drinking?

8. How do you feel the next day after drinking?

As you can see, a lot of these questions are based around when you drink, what you drink, how much you drink, and the feeling alcohol gives you during and after drinking.

Now that you have hopefully answered the eight questions, I am going to show you how I would answer all eight myself. Remember, I have stopped drinking alcohol over a year but just like yourself, I first decided to go sober and ever since then I have just been keeping up with my decision.

Ready?

1. Do you drink after a weekday at work?
- "I don't drink alcohol"

2. Do you drink on weekends?
- "I don't drink alcohol"

3. How many days a week do you drink?
- "I don't drink alcohol"

4. What time of day do you usually drink?
- "I don't drink alcohol"

5. What do you drink?
- "I don't drink alcohol"

6. How much do you drink?
- "I don't drink alcohol"

7. How do you feel when drinking?
- "I don't drink alcohol"

8. How do you feel the next day after drinking?
- "I don't drink alcohol"

To answer the 8 questions above it took 16 seconds total. That's 2 seconds for every question. That's not because I can talk very fast, that's because I recited the same answer to any alcohol-related question that can be thrown at me. "I don't drink alcohol".

This is psychological trick that you can use that works. The way in which this works is by remove the mental energy and willpower required to concoct an answer. Essentially, I'm making it as effortless as possible to refuse a drink. The idea of having a drink or to even open a conversation about the prospects of me drinking is completely removed from my frame of thinking. This works immensely well to fend off family, friends, and colleagues and even yourself.

Most people are averse to conflict – be it physical or conversational. You will be inclined not to say "no" to having a drinking. A lot of us are conditioned to saying "yes" when asked for something.

When you say no, a lot of people may not like it, few will argue against it. However, across humans, we lack an urge to say no. We are too scared and fearful of letting other people down. We cave into imaginary peer-pressure to avoid what we think would be upsetting someone else if we refused to drink alcohol with them.

As a personal trainer, I cannot begin to tell you how many times I have had clients infuriate me because someone bought in cake into the office or their partner returned home with a takeaway, or there was a random birthday for their cousin's sister's brother-in-law's auntie's son, so they had a slice of cake, ate a takeaway or went on a binge drinking episode. Upon questioning them as to why this happened and why there were not following their allocated dieting protocols which they "promised" to commit to, I simply get an immediate waffle of excuses firing at me with them hoping that my would end there.

Please don't get me wrong. I don't subject my clients to psychological or verbal abuse. This conversation between them and I might seem like an interrogation seeking a confession and, in some way, it is. However, I am more interested in getting them to realise how their mistakes can be avoided so that they can turn it into a win-win situation.

Win number 1 is that they avoid eating or drinking something they didn't want to.

Win number 2 is that they remain on track on their goals, avoid relapse and don't face the guilt and remorse that is commonly experienced the next day.

Lastly, win number 3 is that they get better at saying "no" so that they can always remain in control of their decisions in the future without having to bow down to peer-pressure.

This is the same case for drinking alcohol. If you want to quit drinking, you don't need a special supplement, you don't need to keep a log of your alcohol consumption (although that can be useful), you don't need to do anything weird, wonderful or magical. You can quit simply by restricting your vocabulary when it comes to alcohol.

This works incredibly well during social settings. If you are out for dinner with friends and if someone asks you if you'd like a glass of wine. Instead of having to think about if one glass is bad for you or not (we've already discussed this previously), you can just politely decline and say, "No thank you, I don't drink alcohol". As you begin your journey towards a more sober lifestyle, you will get better at these situations. You will not fear people questioning you, you will also formulate better responses with greater confidence such as "no thank you, I'll get a sparkling water today please".

You will know you are on the right side of sobriety once these type of questions is rarely or no longer asked towards you in life. Personally, this took about 6 - 8 months before pretty much everyone in my life got the message and learnt to live with it.

Your family, friends, and colleagues will have now gotten the message very clearly. You have decided to quit drinking alcohol, you have clearly showed great commitment and tenacity towards this goal and show no signs of going back. If we were talking about any other drug here, do you really see your family, friends and loved ones and colleagues encouraging you to restart consuming recreational drugs? I certainly hope not and if your answer is yes, I'd seriously advise on seeking new connections in life.

Just my two cents.

Detoxing Dopamine

We have discussed in great lengths the effects of alcohol and how it plays a role in the release of dopamine in your brain.

It is important to realise that when you begin to quit drinking alcohol, you are removing a source of dopamine in your life. Depending on how much alcohol you used to consume, this might be one of the biggest sources of dopamine or it could fall a lot lower in the things that bring you pleasure in life.

That is why it is important to become very clear with yourself just how much reliant you are on alcohol for brining you joy in your life. If you derive a great deal of joy form consuming alcohol, there will be a void that needs to be fulfilled.

Personally, for myself, I realised that I was using alcohol far too much to bring joy into my life. When I decided to quit drinking, I had to find a means to replace this. A lot of people will look for other quick, easy and cheap joys in life such as eating junk food, smoking, binge watching television, seeking short-term partners and the list goes on.

Whilst each one of these can be distracting enough to prevent you from drinking alcohol again, it is never a smart idea to replace one bad thing with another bad thing.

I chose to commit to 365 days of working out without a rest break. I wouldn't advise everyone to do this because it may not be for them. For me, this was an incredibly beneficial decision to make because it meant that I would get the benefits of working out each day – better energy, more mental clarity, a better-looking body overtime and just feel a whole lot happier and better about life!

The great thing about this is that it also meant I had to be more mindful on my overall nutrition to aid my recovery between workouts since I was planning to not take any days off. This enabled me to replace one bad thing – alcohol, with two positive things – exercising and healthy eating.

The most important part of this decision was the level of commitment. By committing to training every single day, I knew it would be hard work. I did want to make it any harder for myself than I needed it to be. Therefore, if I was to go out drinking, I know I would be suffering the next day with a headache, nausea, tiredness or any other hangover effects from drinking. This made it highly discouraging to want to drink alcohol and interrupt the next day's training.

After a few weeks of being sober and training every single day, I no longer wanted to drink any alcohol. I didn't feel that it would make me anymore happier in life. Instead, I was gaining a lot of the joy in my daily life from exercising. That is because exercise helps to release a lot of endorphins and dopamine – both at neurotransmitters that make you feel good.

Here are a couple of ideas you can use to produce more dopamine without having to use alcohol for the same affect.

- Read books
- Listen to podcasts
- Go for a walk
- Start a new hobby
- Meet up with friends more regularly
- Spend time with your family more regularly
- Play video games instead of going to pubs/ clubs etc.

Any activity that makes you feel good is likely to be secreting dopamine in your brain. I'd suggest you do what you feel is best for you but, if you can get a benefit out of it at the same time, why not?

Deal With Your Problems

After replacing alcohol with another source of dopamine in your life, you may still not be out of the woods when it comes to building a new and more fulfilling life.

I stated earlier how alcohol is often used subconsciously as a crutch to mask away a lot of the problems you face in life. These problems can vary from insecurities, financial, relationships etc. If you are reading this book, the chances are that alcohol has played a big role in your life to some degree. If this is the case, then a lot of the more meaningful things in your life may have been neglected for some time whilst alcohol was at the forefront.

I want to tell you that it is not entirely your fault. Alcohol is a drug, and drugs limit your perception of events and how you perceive your quality of life. However, it is your responsibility to take ownership of your past decisions and to make new decisions which lead to better actions.

I want you to think about five things you would wish for in your life if you could wake up tomorrow and have them all.

What would they be?

Who would you become?

Below, I've left space for you to jot down five wishes that you could wake up to tomorrow.

1.

2.

3.

4.

5.

Here would be my answers before I made the decision to get sober and quit drinking alcohol.

1. To get in the best shape of my life and be at 10% body fat.

2. To spend more time with my parents.

3. To immerse myself in a fulfilling relationship with a life-long partner.

4. To be more present in the moment with day-to-day activities in life.

5. To create a passive stream of income which I can grow to the point I quit my job.

Now imagine what would happen if you had all these things in your life.

How would your life look like?

How would your life it be different?

Would your life be better?

Would you enjoy your life more?

The chances are, if you had all the five things you currently wished for in life, you would be more fulfilled, and you'd never consider the need to drink alcohol ever again. Instead of wishing for these five things to enter your life, it is best that we turn them into goals.

Here is how I would turn my five wishes above into goals that I can work towards.

1. I will reach 10% body fat by the end of 365 days by exercising each day and focusing on eating healthily with defined nutrition targets.

2. Over the next year, I will try to spend at least one evening with my parents and I will try to call or text them more frequently throughout the week.

3. I will make active attempts to date woman and seek to find a partner whose values align with my own and is committed to having a long-term relationship and not just a fling.

4. I will practice mindfulness daily by investing time into reviewing my goals, journaling, meditating and actively listening when engaging in conversations.

5. I will create a new stream of income by attempting ventures such as self-publishing, drop-shipping and other means.

Below, I've left space for you to turn your five wishes into five defined goals that you can work on whilst on your journey of quitting alcohol and becoming sober.

1.

2.

3.

4.

5.

Managing Your Relationships

Lastly, it is important to understand that you are in full control of yourself. It is your life; therefore, it is your decisions that you live up to. Whatever you can control, you can control. Whatever you cannot control, you can at least impact.

Most of the time, alcohol is consumed during social settings. If this isn't the case for you and you usually drink alcohol by yourself, it is important to really investigate how alcohol, dopamine and the affect it has on your mind is playing a role in your life.

Either way, if you drink alcohol in social settings or by yourself, you will experience a barrage of questioning from family, friends and even new people you come by once they find out you have decided to quit drinking alcohol.

You may find that a lot of the people you used to drink with may initially feel upset, concerned or disheartened by your decision because they dread that they will no longer be able to hang out with you anymore. Be prepared to be questioned for the reasoning behind your decision.

However, I do not want you to feel as though you need to ditch your family and friends to quit drinking alcohol. In some cases, yes some of your peers can be part of the reason as to why alcohol has become so prominent in your life, and you may be left with the decision of having to avoid certain people to reach your goal of quitting alcohol for good.

In a lot of cases, your peers will end up supporting your decision because most people genuinely understand that alcohol is not a net-positive on your body, mind and mental health. Most of the time, if you explain your reasoning well to your family, friends, and colleagues, they should be understanding and supportive.

If you want to continue spending social time with whoever it might be in your life, you can do so without having to drink alcohol. Whilst your family and friends are enjoying an alcoholic beverage you are free to drink anything else but alcohol!

This can include water, tea, coffee, soft drinks and even alcohol-free versions of alcoholic beverages.

After going sober, I still hang out with my friends on nights out. I usually start off with an alcohol-free beer or two and then switch over to soda with lime cordial. Yes, it is not that cool to drink alcohol-free beverages and soft drinks but after a few social occasions, no one cares what I'm drinking. At the end of the day, I show up to social events, still engage with my friends like I used to when I was drinking, and no one bats and eyelid at me for it.

It is at the point now that a lot of my friends are highly impressed by it, continue to support my decision, discourage me from even thinking about drinking alcohol and a few are starting to reduce their consumption and even quit themselves. Win-win.

PROBLEMS YOU WILL ENCOUNTER AND HOW TO OVERCOME THEM

"RECOVERY IS ABOUT PROGRESSION, NOT PREFECTION."

— Bill W

Dopamine Withdrawal

One of the biggest problems you will encounter when you are deep on your journey of quitting alcohol is feeling a sense of withdrawal. A lot of people confuse dopamine withdrawal with alcohol withdrawal.

As mentioned previously, genuinely dragonised alcoholics are dependent on alcohol to the extent that if it you immediately remove alcohol from their life, it can lead to death. Alcoholics need professional medical help to taper their alcohol consumption to wean them off it and eventually lead them towards a path of sobriety.

However, for most people who decide to quit alcohol, they may feel some sense of withdrawal symptoms and a craving to drink alcohol again. This is where the possibility of relapsing can take place. It is vitally important to understand that the withdrawal symptoms you may experience from going sober are not a feeling of needing to drink alcohol but instead, a feeling of needing a dopamine release.

When you feel urged to have a drink, you need to stop and think for yourself.

Do you really want to drink alcohol?

The chances are the true answer is no. Instead, you are lacking some form stimulation in life that brings you joy.

If you find yourself in a situation feeling like this, it is best to stop for a few minutes and reflect inwards on yourself. What are you true emotions.

Are you bored?

Are you stressed?

Are you tired?

Are you hungry?

All the above four are negatively associated feelings and the quickest way to overcome them is with a sharp dopamine surge thanks to alcohol.

However, I suggest you do not do that at all. Instead, figure out exactly why you feel an urge to have a drink and address that issue head on.

Bored? – do something fun (not drinking)

Stressed? – meditate, journal, listen to music

Tired? – go to bed early or take a nap

Hungry? – enjoy some nutritious food

Unsupportive Family and Friends

Another problem you may face is the dreaded unsupportive family members and friends. Whilst you and I can hope and pray that our peers have our best intentions at heart, life does not always play out that way and some people can be discouraging even when they don't intend to.

If you have family members or friends who do not respect your decision to quit alcohol and stay sober, it is best to express your decision and reasoning once again. It is also good to ask for support from the people who mean the most to you in your life.

However, neither of these actions lead to a favourable solution, then it might be a good idea to step back and distance yourself from certain individuals in your life before trying to reestablish your relationships and boundaries. It is very important that you set boundaries for your own wellbeing and that those boundaries are respected.

If you find an individual continues to repeatedly disrespect your boundaries then sadly, you have to ask yourself if this individual truly has your best intentions at heart and do you seem them fitting into your life in the future?

Lack of Motivation and Discipline

Lastly, you are going to have periods of time where your motivation to stay sober may take a hit. Sometimes you will feel like you can no longer exercise discipline to keep yourself going.

When you start out on becoming sober, you will be highly motivated. This motivation can be used to build your discipline in refusing to drink any alcohol. If this is done for a long enough period, it no longer requires motivation and discipline for you to not drink alcohol. Essentially, it becomes habitual and a lifestyle.

Decision → Motivation

Motivation → Discipline

Discipline → Habit

Habit → Lifestyle

Ask yourself, where do you fall in this path?

If you are at the discipline → habit stage but feel a sense of relapse coming, perhaps you need to work on changing your disciplines into habits. Moreover, if you are at the motivation → discipline stage, you may want to focus your energy from just feeling highly motivated to applying discipline. This involves learning to say "no" when offered alcoholic drinks and to say "no" to yourself when you are feeling tempted to relapse.

There are many stories of people who quit alcohol and have relapsed. Don't allow yourself to become a statistic. More importantly, understand that people who successfully give up drinking and never go back to it, do so because they have managed to go through all the stages above and reach a point where it is a lifestyle decision.

This is the same for achieving any meaningful change in life. Once you decide, you are motivated to follow through with that decision, the hardest part is exercising the discipline to the point that it turns into a habit. When you get to the point that you habitually do not drink alcohol, all you must do is keep on going and it will become a new lifestyle.

CONCLUSION

"IT'S NEVER TOO LATE TO BE WHAT YOU MIGHT HAVE BEEN."

– George Eliot

Alcohol is a drug, a legal for over a century. However, just because something is legal does not mean it is good for you. We have discussed in length the various way alcohol has a negative impact on your body, mind and mental health.

Primarily, alcohol begins its path to take over your life once it has hooks you in with its powerful ability to induce dopamine secretion. Over a longer period, the feel-good nature of drinking alcohol can turn into an addiction used to attain most of the joy in your life.

After building up a dependence on alcohol it can turn into a subconscious tool to mask the problems you are avoiding in daily life. If this isn't addressed soon rather than later, your life can quickly spiral into something you never intended it to be.

Quitting alcohol is all about regaining control over your decisions and how you choose to seek joy in life. It also requires you to be able to communicate this effectively with your loved ones to gain their support. Ultimately, quitting alcohol provides you the ability to find joy in more meaningful things that surround you in life. It also gives you the opportunity to work on your insecurities and life problems whilst simultaneously chasing your goals.

ABOUT THE AUTHOR

Murad Murad (yes both and first name are the same!) is a personal trainer, physiotherapist, Author and public speaker.

He is obsessed with personal development targeted towards improving discipline, building resilience and reaching a state of equanimity in life.

He has trained and treated multiple clients in his career helping them to accel to greater levels of health and personal wellness.

Murad also regularly engages in public appearances including appearing as a guest on podcasts and performing speeches at schools as well as corporate entities such as Lloyds Banking Group and Payload Studios.

amazon.com/author/muradmurad

www.muradfitness.com

info@muradfitness.com

Instagram: @muradfitness

Printed in Great Britain
by Amazon